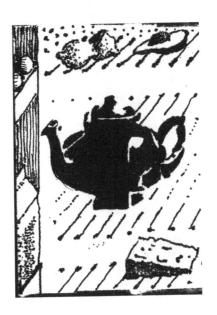

TEAPOT IN THE FRIDGE

POEMS BY

JUDITH BURNLEY

Salamander Street

First published in 2021 by Salamander Street Ltd.
(info@salamanderstreet.com)

Copyright © Judith Burnley, 2021

ISBN: 9781913630829

Printed and bound in Great Britain

10 9 8 7 6 5 4 3 2 1

Contents

Squirrel

When I first met you
You were boyish, eager, bold,
A small red squirrel darting from thought
To swaying thought,
Nibbling away at every new idea.

You hoarded your wisdom in a warm, safe place
And locked the door,
Hiding the entrance with leaves from winters past,
Trusting that memory would turn the key.

And now you are dozing in a darkened room,
Listening and not listening to music you once knew
And to the silence when the music stops.
Wondering now and then what happened to that key
And to the nuggets stored under that tree.

Watching the shadows lengthen as they creep
Up to the chair you sit in, half asleep.

Words

Bit by bit I'm losing you,
The man I loved.
Words that you used to play with joyously
Now float above
That lion's head of yours,
Just out of reach.
The nectarine and the curious peach
No longer tempt you with
Their tastes unknown.
The blossoms of your childhood
Are all blown.
We live now in the moment, fleetingly,
Watching the countdown to Eternity.

Names

What must it feel like
When the names of all the things
You're used to using every day –
Cup, mug, plate, spoon and knife –
Have vanished, or have somehow
Gone astray?

You can still use them,
Eat, drink, wash them up,
Something it pleases you to do,
Yet when I say "Pass me the butter"
You offer me a fork,
Or "Can I have a towel?" you ask
"This?" "This?" or "This?"

No use to talk about it,
Just to hold each other tight,
And kiss.

Clouds

The clouds have character today,
Big fluffy white against the blue,
All those that come in subtle shades of grey,
And ragged, darker ones which threaten rain.

I scan the sky for warnings, but only see
On the insistent screen of my mind's eye
The scan they took of your once brilliant brain,
For there are clouds there, too.

Feathery clouds and indistinct,
But soon they will obscure
So much of all you've known and loved
And worked a lifetime for.

A gust of wind, a sunlit squall
Might chase some clouds away,
But those locked fast inside your head
Are threatening to stay.

Second Childhood

What can I do, when in the street
You stop to play with every child you meet?
What can I say when every dog you see
Is spoken to in Dog, with childish glee?

A squirrel shinnying up a tree,
A pigeon hopping, or a crow on wing
Are given names which have the ring
Of your first Mother tongue,
Those unforgotten sounds.

So on a windy day I fear a kite
Might make you want to join it in its flight
And soar away
Back to the nursery where you used to play
And the bright memories of that long lost day.

Going Gaga

Poor young neurologist, I pity you.
Outside your office in the hospital, a queue
Of gaga oldies sit and wait in hope
That you will conjure up some magic cure
And so confound their terrifying fate.
And all the time you know too well
There's nothing you can do.

Once we all lived in families
With grandpa by the fire in his old chair
And nanny in the kitchen corner, her old lair.
They were 'sixpence short of a shilling'.
They were 'not all there'.
But life went on around them
And no one seemed to care.

Old age can be accepted only by the young.
It's funny and endearing if your time is long,
But if you're coming to the end
There's no way to contain
The pain, the rage, the disgust of decline.
Those bloody chimes at midnight,
Wherefore did they chime?

Growing old gracefully may once have been the aim
But going gaga gently is totally insane.

Don't Stare

Absent minded
Not all there
Not quite normal
Please don't stare.

Three farthings short of a penny
Three shillings short of a pound
Three muffins short of a dozen
Three echoes short of a sound.

Not got all his marbles
Rather lost the plot
A little bit doo-lally
Doesn't know what's what.

One sandwich short of a picnic
Lights on but no one home
Going slightly gaga
Forget his own name soon.

A bridegroom short of a wedding
A baby short of a birth
A coffin short of a funeral
A comedy short on mirth.

The Empty Room

Your mind reminds me of an empty room
Echoing with sounds of long lost revelry.
Once it was richly furnished, subtly lit, and lined
With books you'd read, or you and friends
Had writ. Treasures from all your travels.
Paintings that glowed.
It was a haven where you could retreat
And find the strength there to defeat
The perils of the brutal world outside:
A place of safety and a source of pride.
Perhaps it is a blessing that you cannot tell
How bleak and bare it has become – a shell
On a deserted beach, a spring dried up, a well
Where no stone reaches water
For the knell rings only in my head, not yours,
Reaching you muffled and remote as where you dwell
On distant, uninhabitable shores.

Patience

I walk on eggs now, every single day
But I've no patience to repeat
The third of fourth time, everything I say.
I'm only human.

In the end I raise my voice,
Speak loud and clear and slowly to your face
As if you were a child. Bad move.
You're angry and you shout "Don't shout at me!"
And go into a huff.
Huffs may last several days.

I try to soothe, apologise, placate,
While inwardly I'm raging at my fate
And longing, simply, just to run away.

But underneath all this, love lingers.
I still care.
However hard it gets, I know
I have to stay.

Where?

This is the hardest of all things to bear
The lost, bewildered look, the mute despair
The fear that cries out where has it gone
The me, my Self, the man I used to be?
You must know where it is, you always do.
You'll find it for me in another room,
Under the bed, or in an old armchair
And give it back to me.
Of course I will, I long to say.
And then you stare all a long afternoon
At the first page of a book you wrote yourself
But cannot understand a word.
There's nothing I can do
Except be there.

Bored Rigid

'Oh, it's a tragedy,' they said. 'you'll see,
You'll have to watch as he declines.
You're losing him, it's like a curse,
And there's no remedy – it will get worse.'
But what they didn't tell me was
Just how bored I'd be.
They should have known.
You would be if you got
Some twenty-seven repetitions
Before tea.

Over and over and over again
The same bitter story,
The same sour refrain.
They were black and you were white,
They were wrong and you were right.

Shut up, shut up, you want to say,
I've heard it all before
But if you don't fake interest
And stifle that big yawn
The anger will erupt again
And you'll be cowering in your chair
In full force of the storm.

Pompeii

Your anger erupts, a live volcano
White hot your ire,
Scarlet is your face and torso
Lava from a terrifying fire.

Your screams assail me like rocks thrown.
You shout resentments, settling old scores.
Nothing that ever hurt you is forgotten
But burns and blisters in the molten pyre.

I'm frozen in a corner where
The thumping of my own heart beat
Sounds fearful, like the tramp of marching feet.
One day they'll find me here, preserved in terror,
And I won't speak.

Alone

How can I learn to live like this
Alone, but not alone?
The presence of a hollow man
Looms like a mighty monolith
Far weightier than stone.
For like a stone he cannot speak
And like a child his eyes entreat
And though I groan, I also weep
For what can never be.

Where has it gone, the joy, the fun
The laughter? And the warm glow
That always lingered after?
Now we must cherish every loving look
Before the story's ended
And we close the book.

Escape

I dreamed last night
That I had run away.
I was out in the open
Free as the air
Just as I used to be.
I could read, sleep and think,
Stare at the changing light,
Talk freely to my friends until
The middle of the night.
I could watch old films
Dance to old tunes:
I could be me.
Then I awoke and you
Were snoring gently, as you do
And I was trapped again
By that old siren call:
The childlike neediness of you.

Teapot

Today I found the teapot in the fridge
Complete with tea bag and the dark brown dregs of tea.
This is a first.
It might be knickers next,
Or something worse.
You've got to laugh.
"You put the teapot in the fridge," I said.
"What next?
Perhaps I'll find the kippers in the bed."
But now it's only I who laughs, and you,
Whose wit was legendary,
Sing gently to yourself
Some unforgotten tune.

What Now?

Things have got so serious now
I don't know what to do.
Little of what I say these days
Is understood by you.
Words have detached themselves from meaning,
Fallen off the tree
Like leaves in winter's winds.
Repeating only makes you cross.
Explaining's hard to do. What now?
Will we, who made such joyful music
With the words we loved, live now
Inside a grey and silent world?

Recognition

Every day you say you've never seen
This dress before.
Time was you noticed everything
I wore, how my hair fell
Whether I was tired or unwell.
What do you see now when you look at me?
The worried woman, or the girl
I used to be?
One day you might not know
This face is mine.
But I will still know yours
And love it still.
I dread that time.

High Chair

You sit at table like a child in his high chair.
You hold a spoon aloft.
You turn your head to left and then to right.
Look at me! Look at me!
I've got a spoon.
It's Power.
You won't take it away from me.

And yesterday inside a busy shop
You'd found the juice you like and held it up
For all to see.
Two women passing were amused.
You've got a good one there, they nodded,
Reassuringly.
They saw a man in his late seventies.
They couldn't know
That you are only three.

And when you run to other babies in the street,
You simply want to play with them.
They understand.
But their young mothers, always in a rush
Hurry them away, and you look after them
With a bewildered look.

Is there no future for the child
Trapped in an old man's body?
No one knows.
And so you stand and stare along the street,
Abandoned and alone.

Grace

Today a child you'd never seen before
A tiny boy of not yet two
Ran with his arms outstretched across the grass
To you.

You picked him up and held him face to face.
He kissed your cheek.
And then you gently put him down.
You did not speak.

No words
Could ever say how sweet that moment was
In all its unexpected grace.

Free Play

What does it matter if you're not all there
When you're as happy as you were today?
Life a surprising breakfast tray
Of sweets and treats you've never seen before.
Or so you say.

A petal swaying in the breeze
Caught on a cobweb thread so fine
It is invisible. You are entranced.
You don't know what a cobweb is
Or why the petal swings like this.
You cannot tell a petal from its flower.
You cannot tell a moment from an hour.

"It's playing by itself, don't touch.
I want to play with it," you say.
"I want to watch."

Long may you play.

Taste

The words for chair and table have long gone, and yet
You sit down facing me each day all smiles, and eat
But whether what you taste is fish or meat,
The same or different from the meal of yesterday
I cannot tell. Nor do I know
If taste and smell exist without their names
Though you say 'yum'
Like the small child you have become.
So all I can do is cook with love and flair
To make these shadowed days less hard to bear.

Routine

Everyday you have to go to the same shop
By the same route. We may not need a thing
But you must stick to your routine
So that you still feel useful in the world
Just as you still insist on washing up
Imperfectly, in that old-fashioned way
Ignoring my trusty dish washing machine.
And so I make a shopping list.
You go through it six times.
Marmite's a mystery. I show you the empty jar.
You're baffled, so I cross it off.
And what is meant by this word 'tin'?
A can, a container. I show you a tin of soup.
You're sure to come back with something
In a box. Something I never use.
'They helped me in the shop,' you say.
'They were so nice,' And I'm left puzzling.
What can I cook to use up so much rice?

Some Nights

Some nights you throw yourself across the bed
And your arms flail about.
You're in a fight, you scream and shout,
But still you're fast asleep. I dare not touch or
Try to wake you – I'd be inside the dream
And that, of course, could mean
That you'd hit me.
And so I edge myself out of the bed,
Switch on the bedside light, and wait
For all this unleashed violence to abate.

Last night you threw yourself on to the floor.
The crash awakened me. 'Are you alright? I called.
You were confused.
Where were you? What was going on?
You were not hurt at all.
Your body bounced, just like a baby's would.

It seems these nightmares are of childhood fears.
The worst was when I heard your voice
At three or four years old, trying so hard
To sing along – a good little boy in kindergarten
class,
But failing not to choke on your own tears.
The sound of that has haunted me for years.

Lost

You wander, every day, from room to room
Searching for something you can never find.
How can I tell you that it's not your glasses
Or your pen you've lost –
It is your one and only mind.

Who knows what memory is, or where it's found,
In eyes, ears, fingertips,
In clear blue skies, or buried underground?

We reach for it, we dig for it
But we can never hold it warm and safe,
Nor ask it what is false and what is true.
It vanishes, and takes away with it
The rare, the unexpected, the unique,
The taste and smell
Of the essential you.

Shell

I miss you more than when you were away
I miss you more now every single day
And yet you're here
You're standing near
Warm to the touch and still so dear.

But where has the essence of you gone
That complex mix of spicy flavours
The jumble of the right and wrong
The ideas going for a song
That won you friends and favours?

You're like a specially treasured shell
Loved for its subtle coils and colours,
One which, held fast against the ear
Makes waves on a far distant shore
Sound magically near.

It whispers low so only you can hear
Nothing but love and nearness
Can banish fear.

No Hold

How slippery your hold upon the world
Is now, when names and shapes of things
All fall away. You must be terrified
To know you cannot grasp
The ordinary tools of everyday
And are condemned to watch
As the once brilliant colours of your life
All drain to grey.
Your yesterdays are gone
In one small curl of smoke
And as for your tomorrows
There's a closing down,
A coming of the night
No power we can call on
Can revoke.

Quicksilver

Every day there comes a moment when
I know I can't go on like this –
I can't pretend
That you are who you used to be.
And then
I long for what is lost.

Where is it now, the once quicksilver wit?
All gone the mimicry, the mockery, the song,
The silly ancient jokes, the laughter,
And that warm glow which always lingered after.

We live in shadow now, and so
It may be just as well
You don't remember how the light
Once spun about your head
And cast a spell.

Evensong

Walking together in the sloping evening sun
Watching the green intensify
Before the shadows fall
And trees turn black against the fading light,
Bracing themselves before the coming night.

Sitting together at the table, candles lit
And relishing the taste of each titbit,
Old jokes, old songs, old memories awry,
Then, suddenly, your eyes are fixed on me
With such a look I cannot turn away.

This is our ordinary life, the life of every day
Til the dawn breaks and shadows flee away.

No Way Back

I am lost, I am lost, you want to say.
I want to go home
I don't know the way.

I want to go back now
I want to be me
You know – the person
I used to be.

Where is he now?
Where can he be?
Can I ever go back
To the man who was me?

Pooh

When the person you love
Has lost his mind
Can't find a word
Of any kind
The what and the wherefore
The why and the who
Who do you send for?
You send for Pooh.

Pooh is a bear of little brain
Thinking for him is quite a strain
But over and over and over again
He comes out with something
True.

And when he's finished guzzling honey
He's sticky and licky and very
Funny.
No better cure for night's despair
Than a battered, one-eyed, cuddly
Bear.

Why You Wander All Night Long

In the last days of my mother
Her small, childlike feet
Would endlessly strive
For the edge of the bed
To escape, to stand up, to say
Look, I'm still here
I can move: I still thrive.

So now when you won't lie still in your bed
But wander the corridors all night long
I know what you're saying:
I am not yet dead.
I can move, I am upright,
I'm restless, alive
And my instinct's still good:
I will fight the good fight
Searching night's terrors
For a last glimpse of light.

Dead

I am dead, you said
And I know it's true
For the person I'm looking at
Is not you.

The bewildered look
The hurt in your eyes
The anger which makes you
Strike at your thighs

Harder and harder, until it hurts.
This animal here. Not me, not me.
Where is the person
I used to be?

You wander through rooms
Which used to be home
As if lost in space
And entirely alone.

Where will I sleep?
In a ditch? In a lair?
Cold, cold in the ground
And you won't be there.

And then you accuse me:
You! You're not dead!
You move to hit me
That moment I dread.

I make no answer.
What can I say?
I'm guilty as hell
I'm alive, if not well.

Where will I sleep?
In a ditch? In a lair?
Cold, cold in the ground
And you won't be there.

Letting Go

How can I let you go
Into such darkness
Frightened
And all alone.

Can't I be Orpheus
Searching the underworld
Calling
Look, darling, I'm here
And I'm bringing you home.

You turn then to follow me
Into the light.
I'm forbidden to look
But somehow I see
You've become spectral thin
So slight, so slight
A shadow of yourself
That cannot be
Exposed to the world
In the glare of daylight.

I weep.

How can I treasure who you were
How keep the memory alive
When you must sleep here in the dark
Alone
As I retreat?